What Happens Next?

DEALING WITH LIFE CHANGES

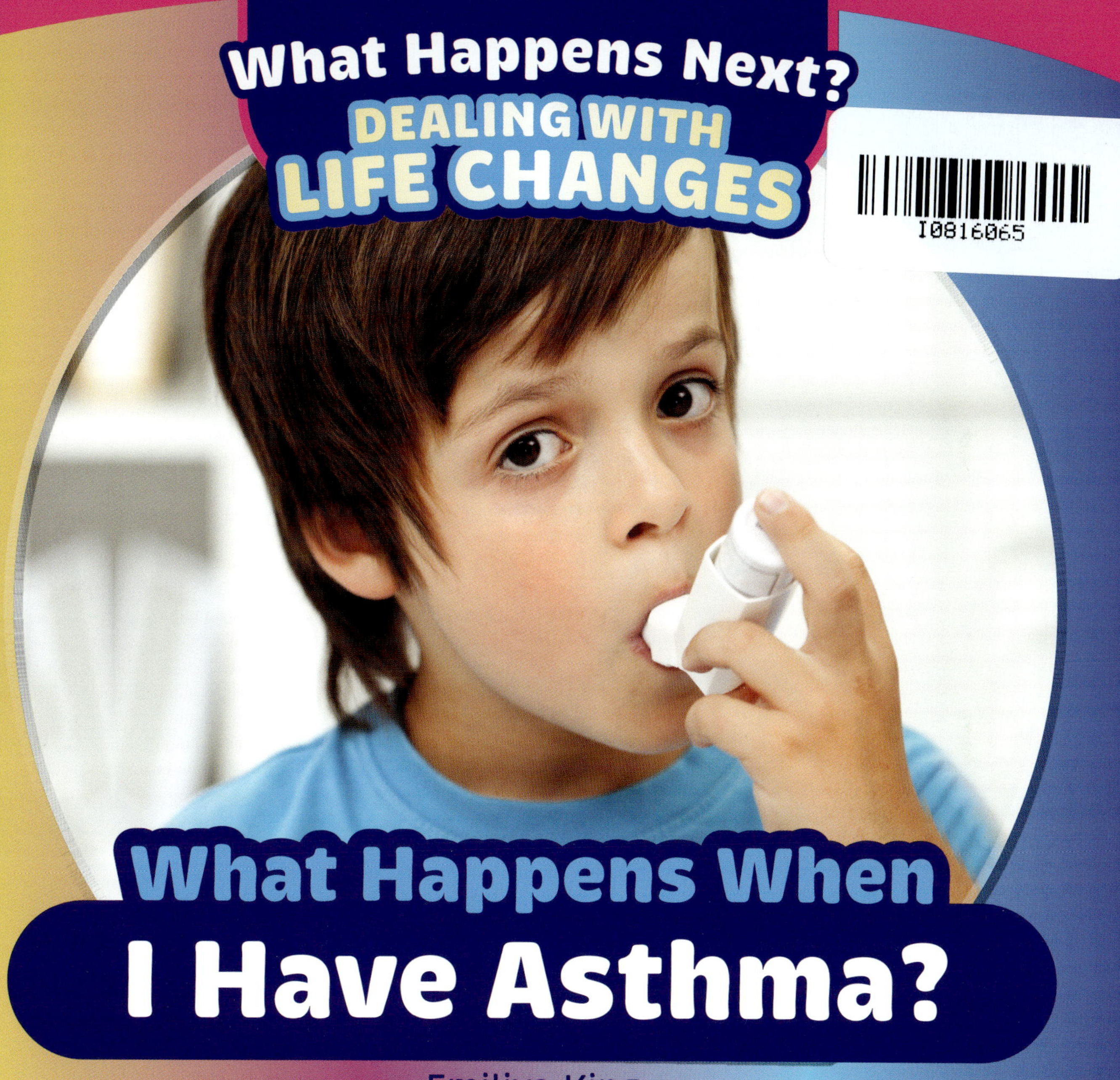

What Happens When I Have Asthma?

Emiliya King

PowerKiDS press.

Published in 2026 by The Rosen Publishing Group, Inc.
2544 Clinton Street, Buffalo, NY 14224

First Edition

Editor: Caitie McAneney
Book Design: Leslie Taylor

Photo Credits: Cover Ilike/Shutterstock.com; p. 5 PeopleImages.com - Yuri A/Shutterstock.com; p. 7 Prostock-studio/Shutterstock.com; p. 9 Yurii_Yarema/Shutterstock.com, (inset) CLUSTERX/Shutterstock.com; p. 11 Peakstock/Shutterstock.com; p. 13 antoniodiaz/Shutterstock.com; p. 15 Prostock-studio/Shutterstock.com; p. 17 T.Vyc/Shutterstock.com; p. 19 Laboko/Shutterstock.com; p. 21 bubutu/Shutterstock.com, (inset) Alexander Gordeyev/Shutterstock.com.

Cataloging-in-Publication Data
Names: King, Emiliya.
Title: What happens when I have asthma? / Emiliya King.
Description: Buffalo, NY : PowerKids Press, 2026. | Series: What happens next? dealing with life changes| Includes glossary and index.
Identifiers: ISBN 9781499452518 (pbk.) | ISBN 9781499452525 (library bound) | ISBN 9781499452532 (ebook)
Subjects: LCSH: Asthma–Juvenile literature. | Asthma in children–Juvenile literature.
Classification: LCC RA645.A83 K46 2026 | DDC 616.2'38025–dc23

Manufactured in the United States of America

CPSIA Compliance Information: Batch #CSPK26. For Further Information contact Rosen Publishing at 1-800-237-9932.

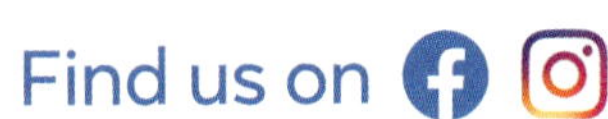

CONTENTS

What Is Asthma?

Do you ever find it hard to breathe? Do you feel short of breath when you try to run, bike, or play sports? Everybody feels short of breath sometimes, especially when they're exercising very hard. But people with asthma may feel this way often—and much worse than others.

Asthma is a **chronic** illness, or one that lasts for a long time or a lifetime. People with asthma have airways that become swollen, narrow, or full of **mucus**. That makes it hard to breathe.

Your Point of View

Nearly 5 million U.S. kids have asthma. It's one of the most common chronic illnesses in children.

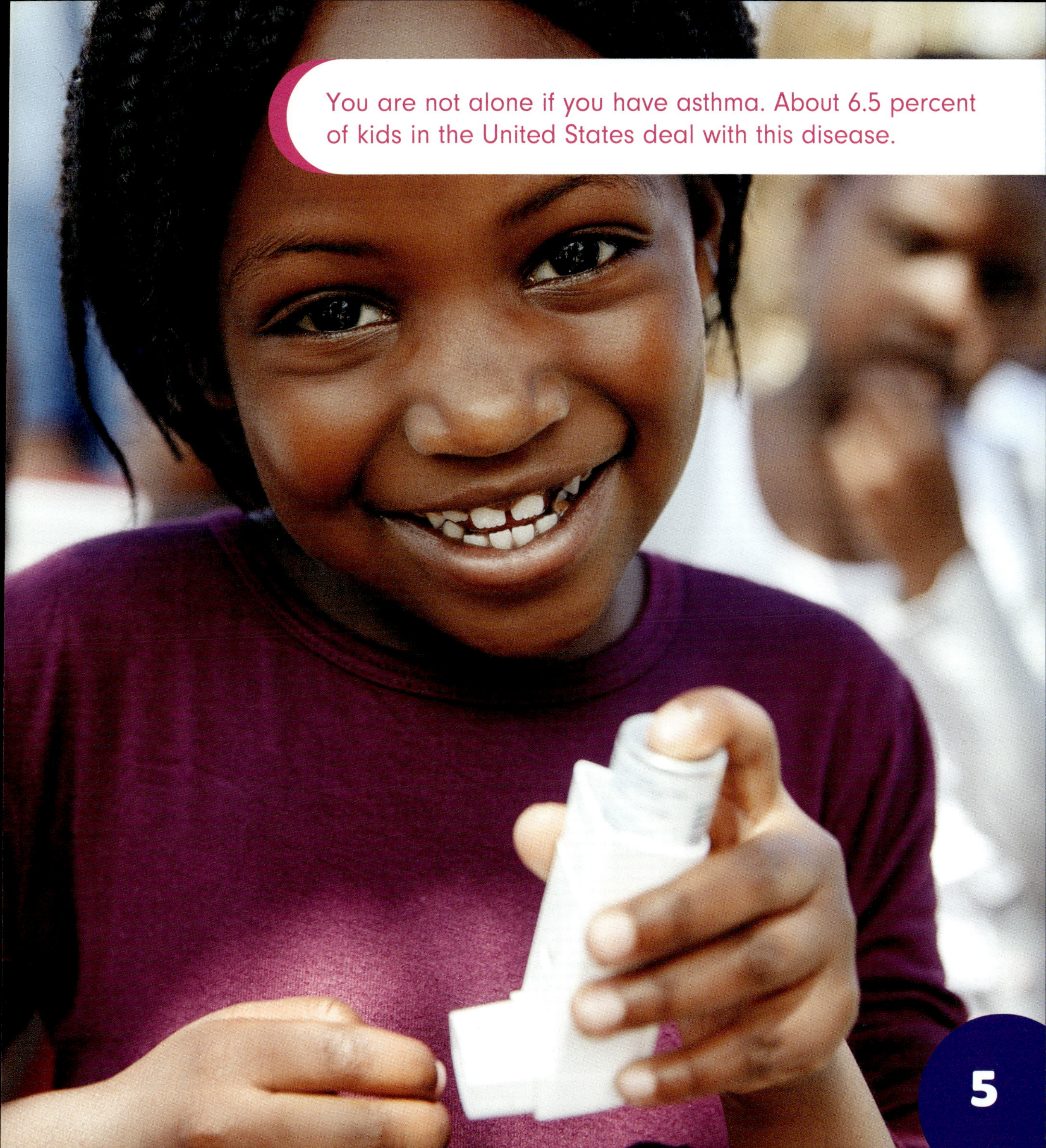

You are not alone if you have asthma. About 6.5 percent of kids in the United States deal with this disease.

Hard to Breathe

When your airways feel **constricted**, it's hard to breathe. You may also cough or wheeze. Wheezing is the sound that air makes when it's moving through narrowed airways. It might sound like a whistle. A flare-up of these **symptoms** is called an asthma attack.

It can be very scary to be unable to catch your breath during an asthma attack. You may start to feel worried, and try to breathe faster, which can cause panic. You may feel like you can't control your breathing.

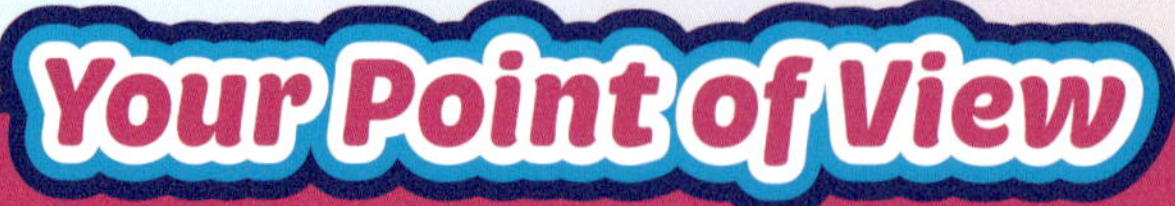

Some asthma **triggers** are **allergies**, pollution in the air, weather, exercise, and **stress**.

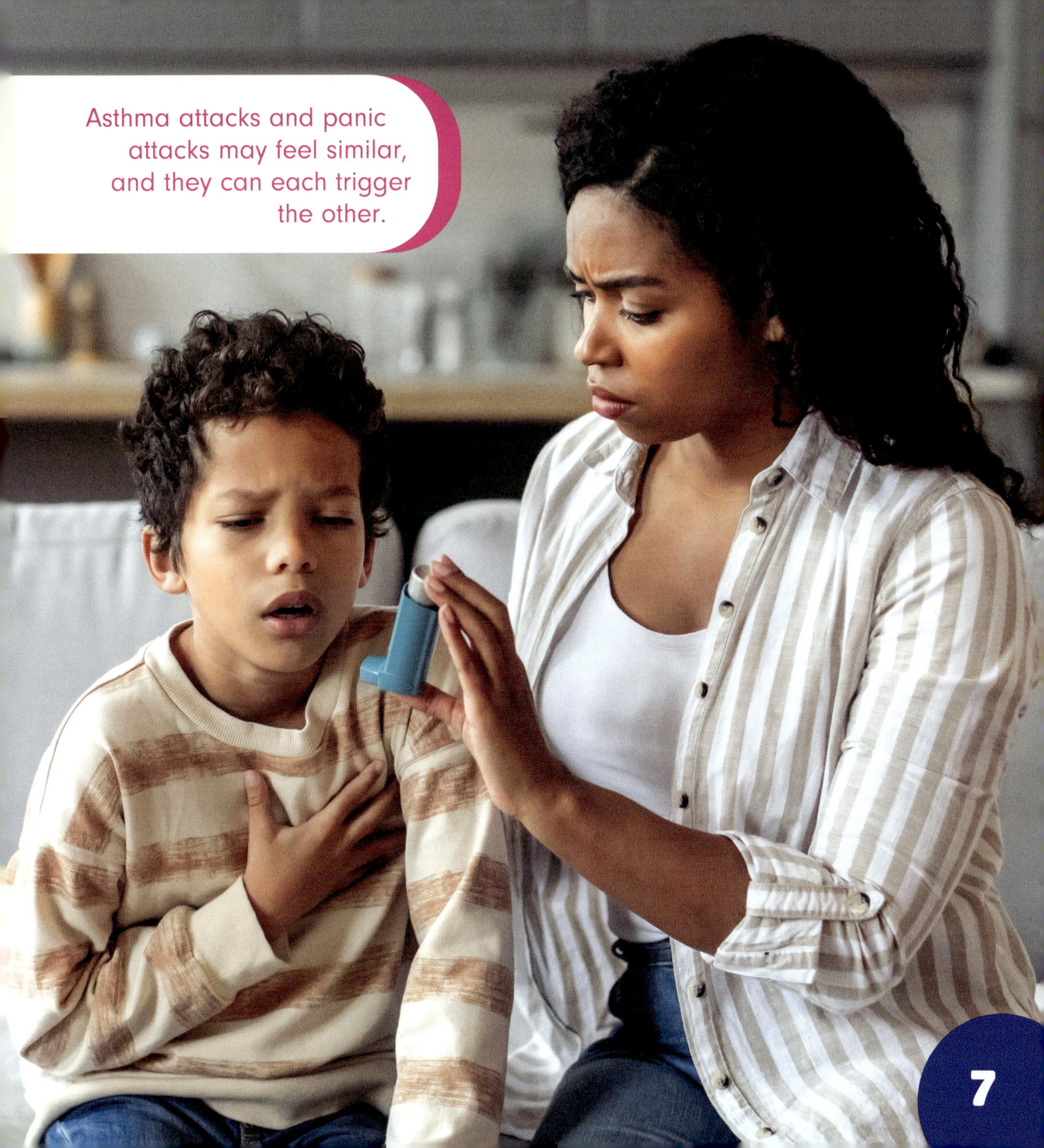

Asthma attacks and panic attacks may feel similar, and they can each trigger the other.

The Respiratory System

Learning more about how breathing works can help you deal with your asthma. The respiratory system is how your body breathes. Breathing supplies the body with oxygen from the air.

Air goes into the body through the nose or mouth, then it moves down the trachea, or windpipe. It branches out into two bronchi, which feed the air into the lungs. The bronchi are like branches of a tree, which divide into smaller branches until they end in tiny air sacs.

Your Point of View

The air sacs at the end of bronchi are called alveoli, and their job is to send oxygen to the blood.

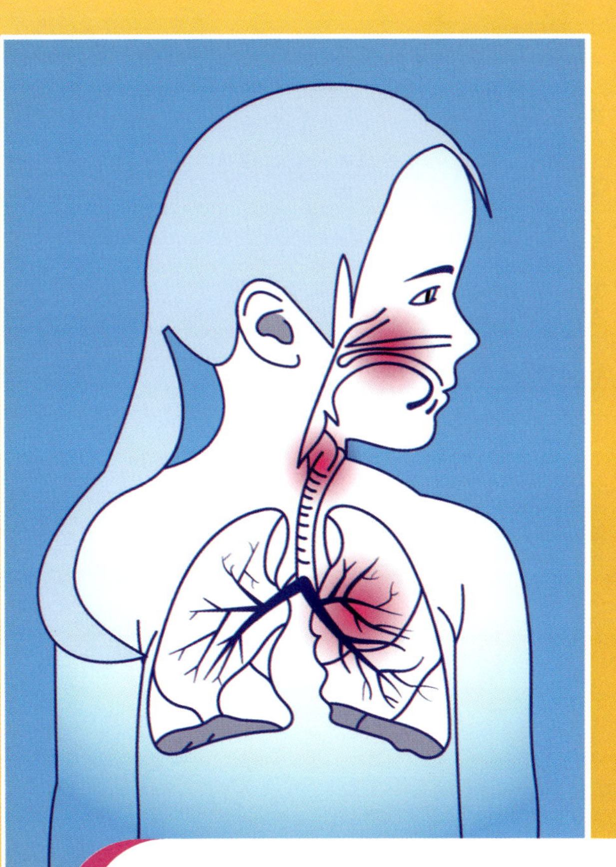

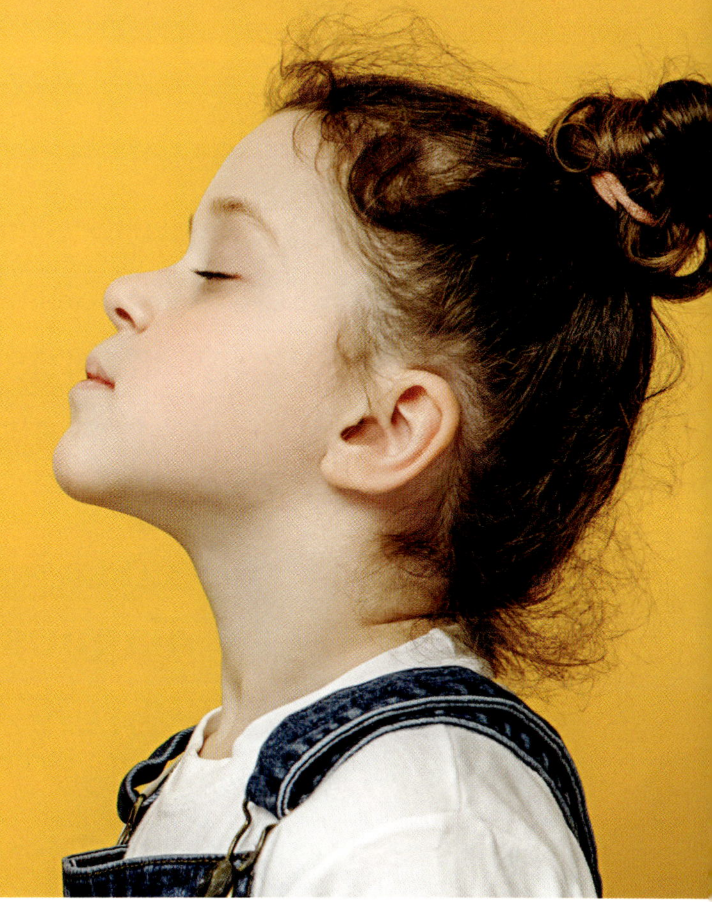

Breathing in, you take in oxygen to help your body work. Breathing out, you let out a harmful waste product called carbon dioxide.

Do You Have Asthma?

If you have asthma, your airways are **inflamed**. That means the path of air to the lungs is blocked. This can be true even if you don't have symptoms. However, when something triggers the airways to become more inflamed or filled with mucus, it can cause an asthma attack.

A doctor can **diagnose** your asthma. They will ask about your symptoms. Then, they'll use a special tool called a spirometer. You breathe into it, and it measures the speed of the airflow.

Spirometers can tell doctors how well your lungs are working.

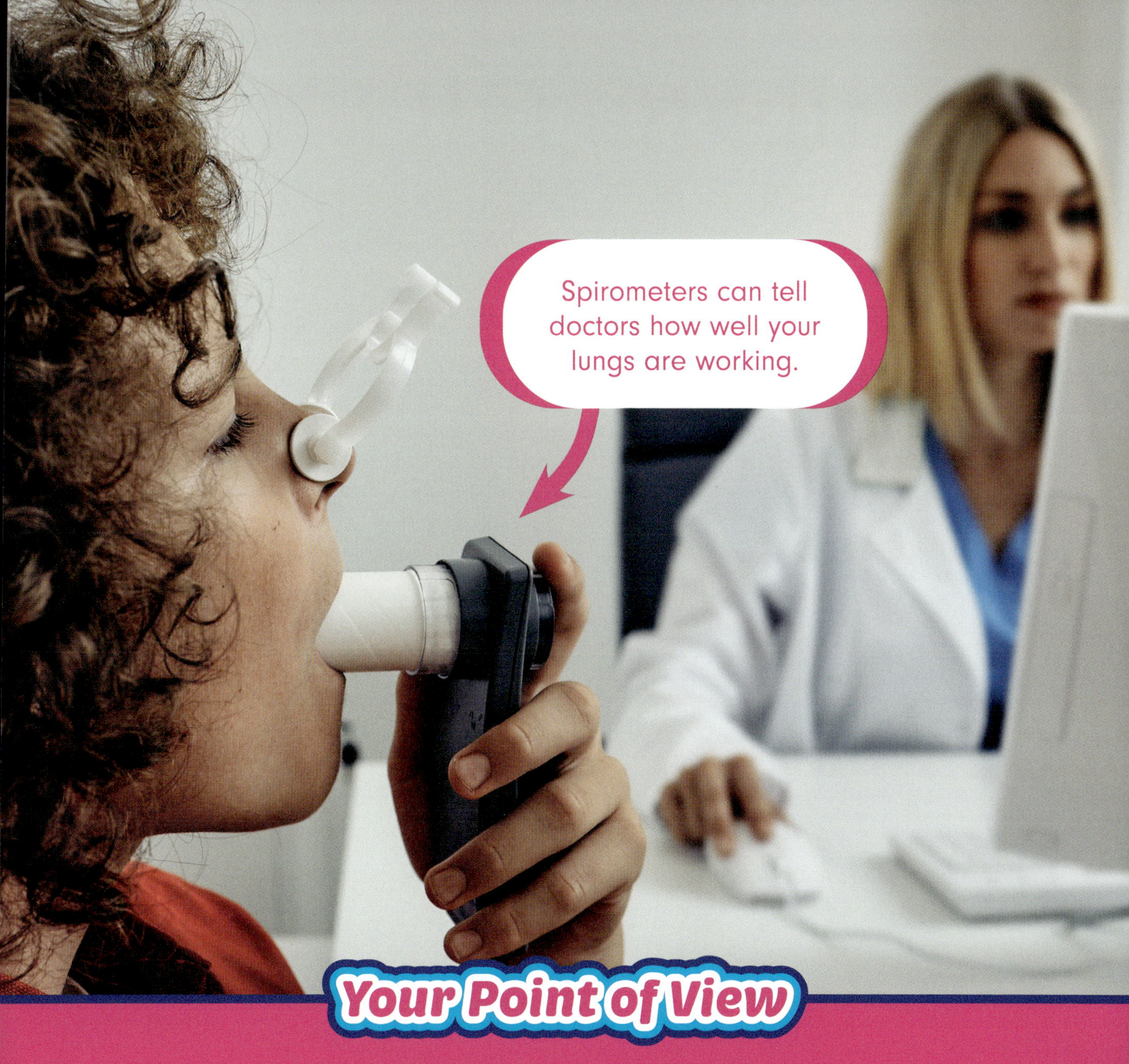

Your Point of View

Asthma seems to run in families. You are more likely to have it if other people in your family have it.

To the Rescue

Once you've been diagnosed with asthma, a doctor can give you special medicine to help you. Some kids take medicine every day that makes their airways less inflamed. Another medicine is taken in an emergency, which is sometimes called a "rescue" medicine. It helps the muscles around the airways relax.

Most asthma medicines are breathed into the lungs in a mist. Inhalers are common tools for taking in asthma medicines. Some kids use their inhalers before exercise or when they feel short of breath.

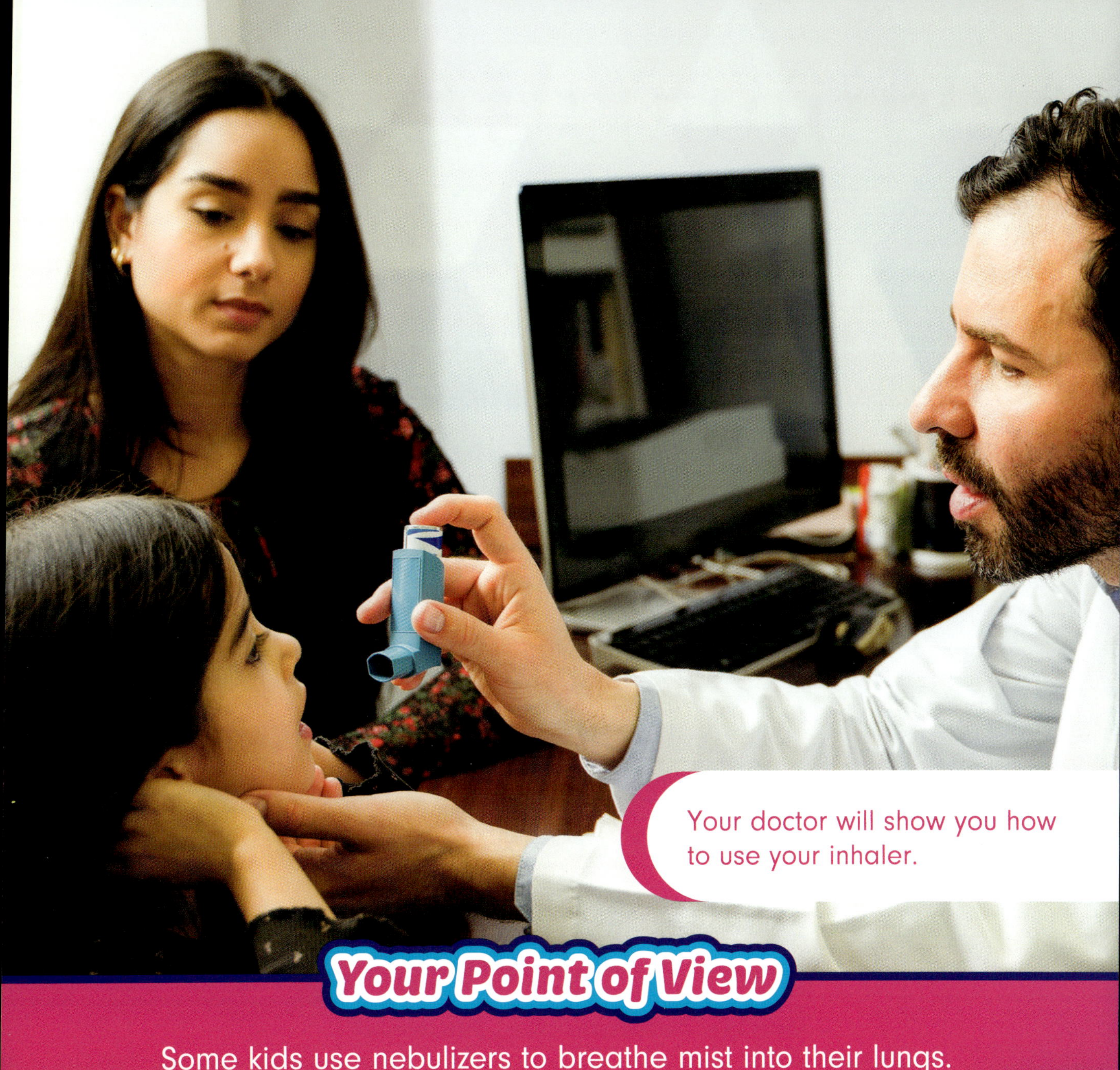

Your doctor will show you how to use your inhaler.

Your Point of View

Some kids use nebulizers to breathe mist into their lungs. Nebulizers cover the mouth and nose and send a medicine-filled mist into the lungs.

Asthma Attack 101

Your doctor will give you an action plan in case of an asthma flare-up. During asthma attacks, you may start coughing and feel like your chest is heavy or tight. It may be hard to get air into the lungs. Take your medicine as your doctor has instructed. Rest your body until the symptoms go away.

In a severe attack, you may have trouble speaking or breathing even if you're sitting still. If your lips start to turn blue or you get **drowsy**, you'll need emergency help. Someone should call 911.

Your Point of View

Some asthma action plans are color coded. Green zone means you're doing well, yellow zone means symptoms are getting worse, and red zone is an emergency.

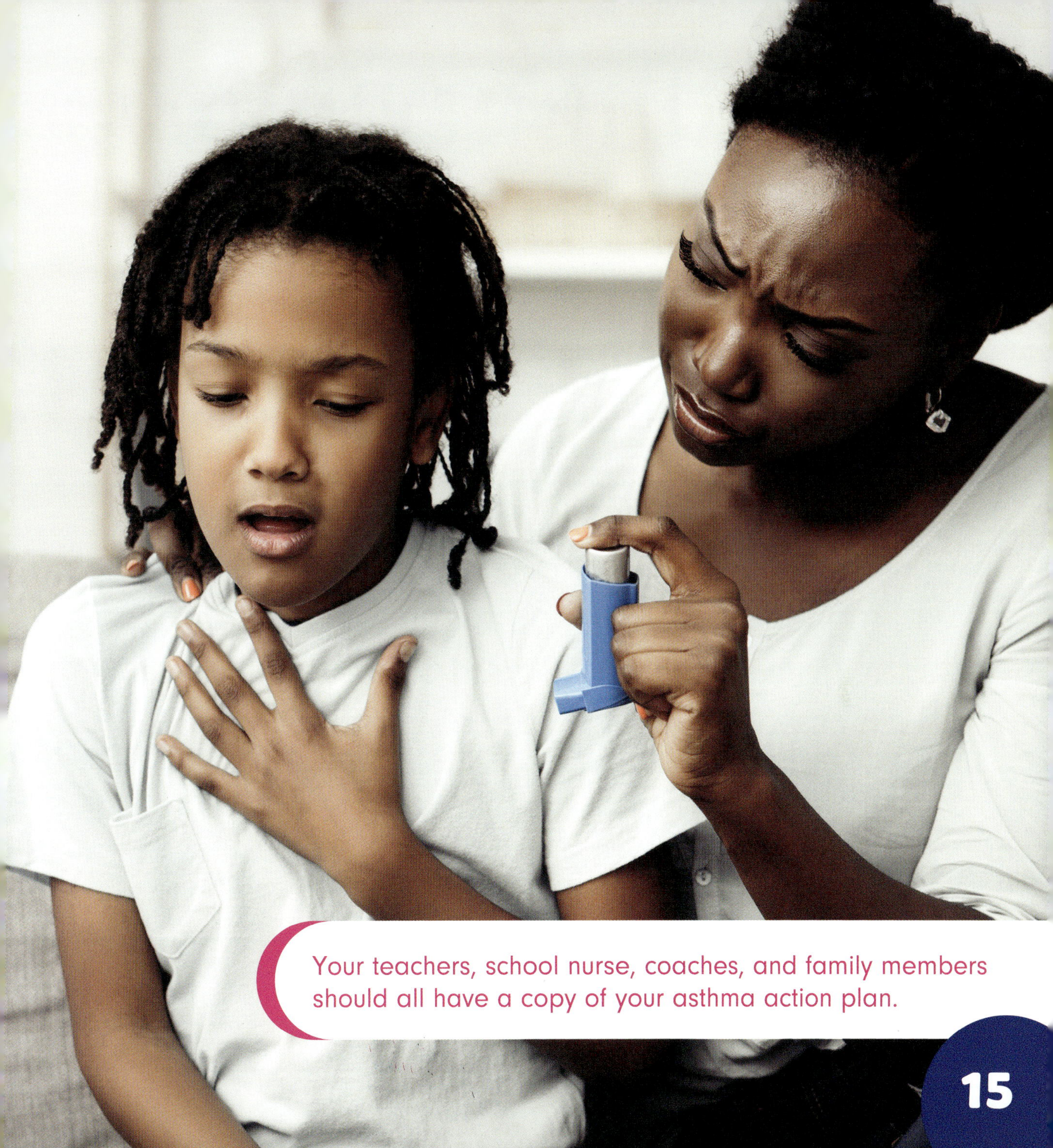

Your teachers, school nurse, coaches, and family members should all have a copy of your asthma action plan.

Avoiding Triggers

An asthma attack can be triggered by things in your **environment**, as well as stress and illness. If you have asthma, you should be extra careful about getting sick. A cold or the flu can make your symptoms worse.

Pollution in the air, such as smoke or smog, can trigger asthma symptoms. If you are allergic to things like mold or pollen, try to avoid them as much as possible. Stay inside when the weather or pollen count make it hard to breathe.

Your Point of View

Emotions are normal and healthy! However, bouts of crying or laughing can trigger an asthma attack.

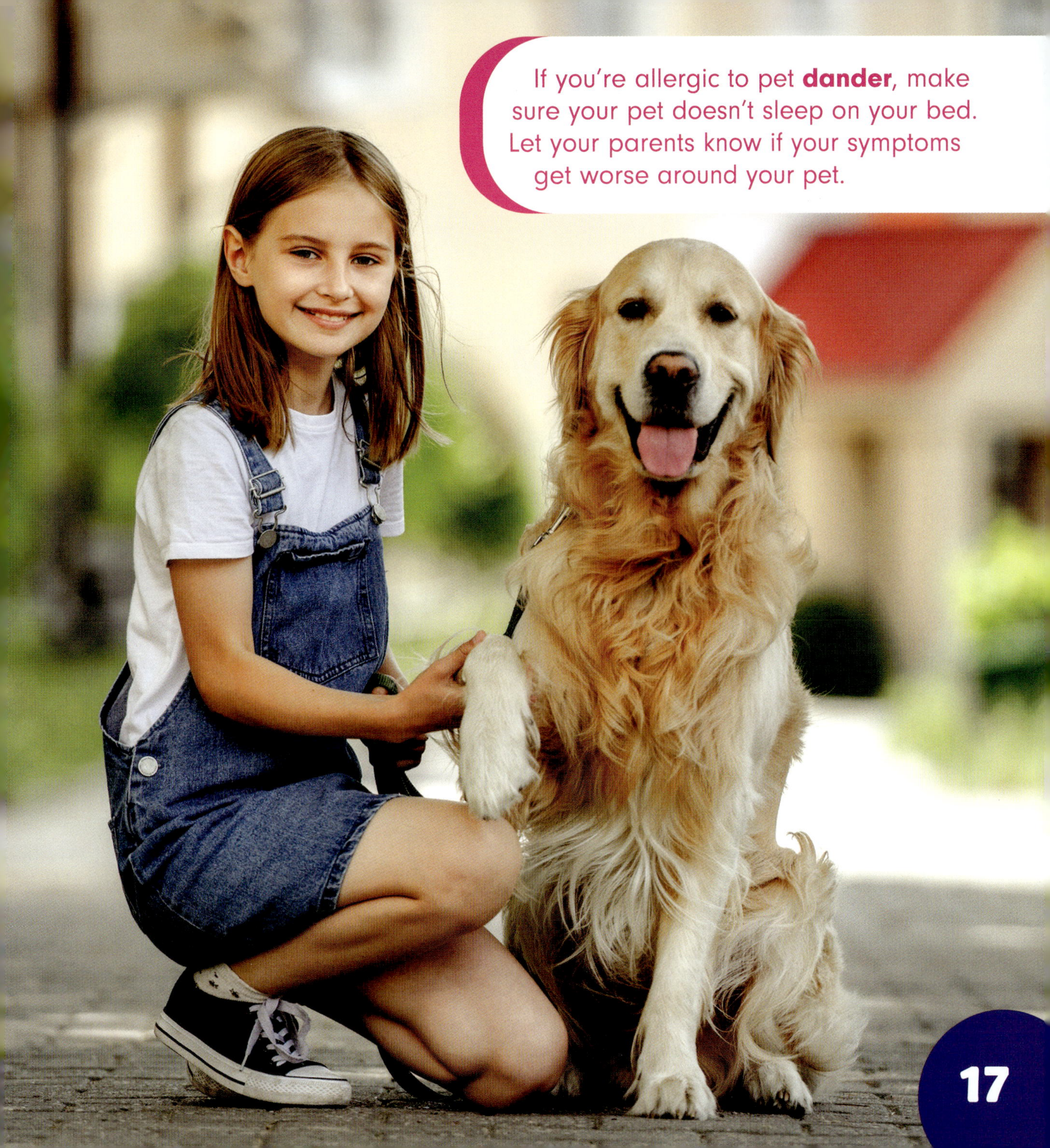

If you're allergic to pet **dander**, make sure your pet doesn't sleep on your bed. Let your parents know if your symptoms get worse around your pet.

Asthma on the Go

You might feel nervous about having an asthma attack while at school, playing sports, or out and about. Make sure the adults in charge know about your asthma action plan and keep your inhaler at the ready. Then you will be well cared for.

Exercise is a common asthma trigger, so sports can make some kids with asthma extra nervous. However, that doesn't mean you should stay still all the time. In fact, moving your body allows your lungs to grow stronger, which can help your asthma.

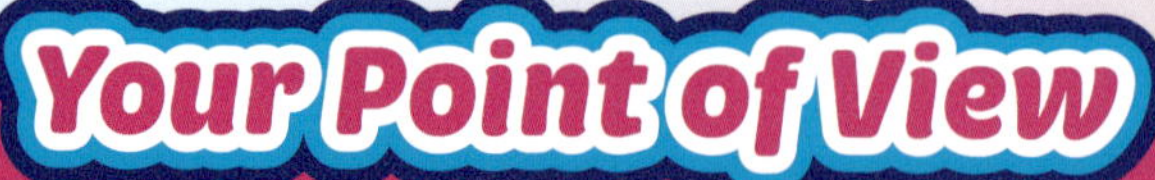

You can carry your inhaler in a purse, bookbag, or sports duffel bag.

You can use an attachment called a spacer, which holds the medicine in place so you can breathe it in easier.

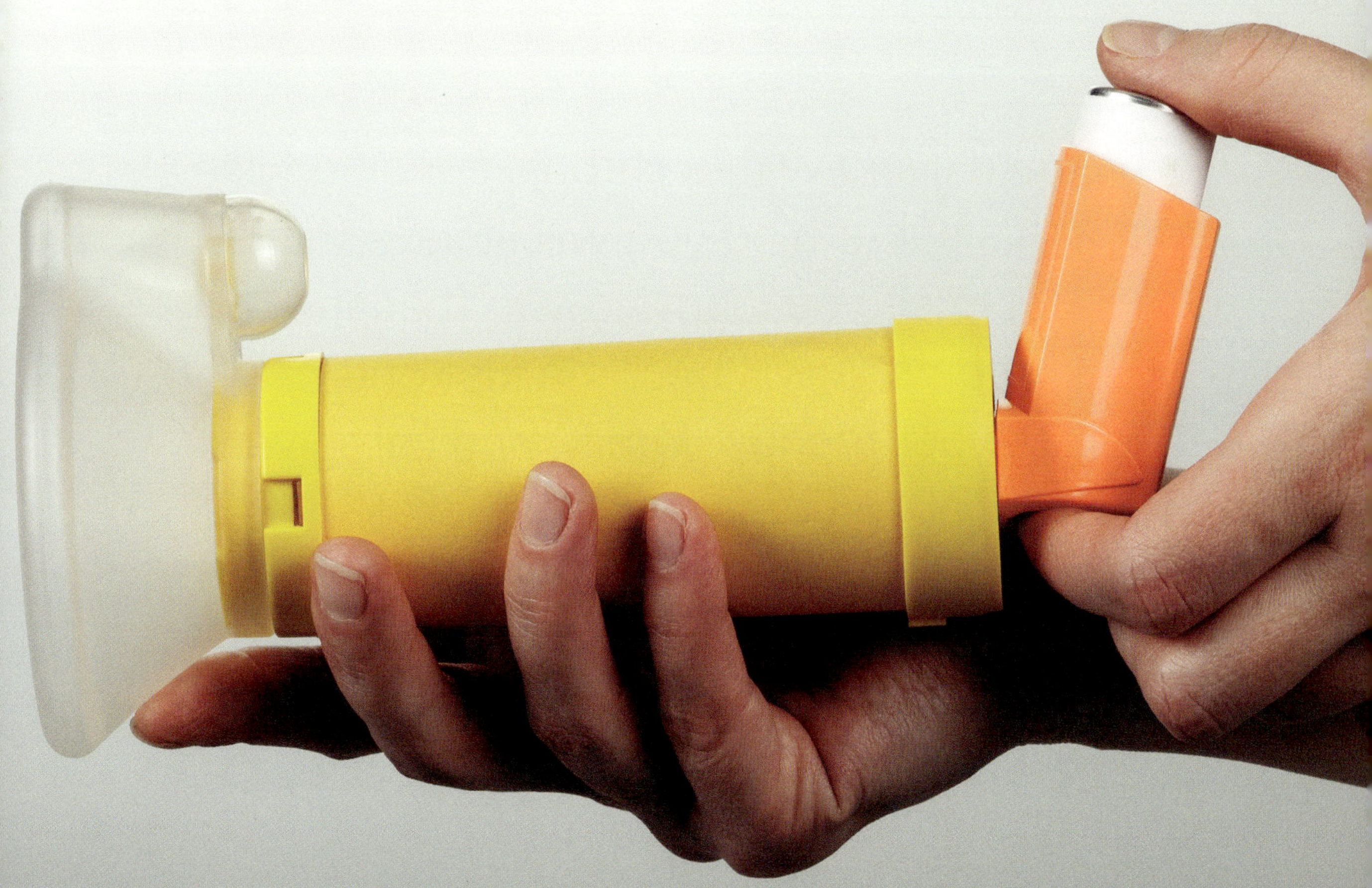

You Can Do Anything!

It's hard living with a chronic condition like asthma. It's something you will always think about. But once you learn how to manage your symptoms, it will become just one part of life. Talk to your friends, family, and caregivers about any worries or emotions you feel.

Some famous athletes have managed asthma even while breaking records. David Beckham, a famous soccer star, has been open about having asthma and using an inhaler when he needs it. You can do anything that anyone else can do!

Your Point of View

Some people have asthma symptoms their whole life. For others, their symptoms get much better as they grow older.

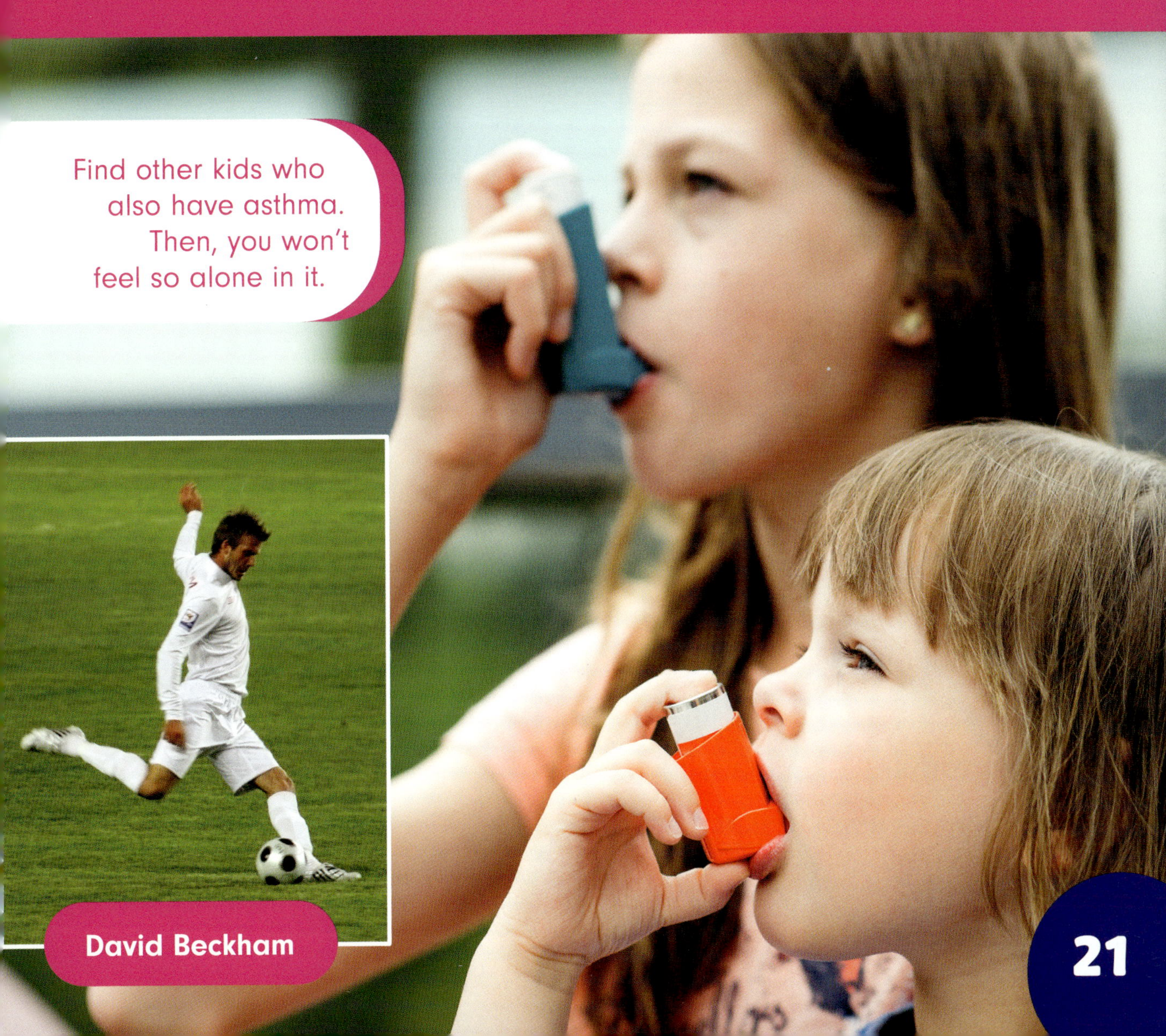

Find other kids who also have asthma. Then, you won't feel so alone in it.

David Beckham

Glossary

allergy: A bad bodily reaction to certain foods, animals, or surroundings.

chronic: Continuing or occurring again for a long time.

constrict: To tighten.

dander: Very small scales from hair, feathers, or skin that may be allergenic.

diagnose: To identify a disease by its signs and symptoms.

drowsy: Very tired.

environment: The natural world in which a plant or animal lives.

inflamed: Having a bodily response to injury in which heat, redness, pain, swelling, and more than the usual amount of blood are present in the area affected.

mucus: A thick, sticky fluid that helps trap dust and other particles.

stress: Something that causes strong feelings of worry.

symptoms: A sign that shows that someone is sick.

trigger: Something that sets off another thing.

For More Information

Books

Mather, Charis. *Asthma Attack*. Minneapolis, MN: Bearport Publishing, 2023.

McClure, Leigh. *The Respiratory System*. Buffalo, NY: Scientific American Educational Publishing, 2025.

Websites

Asthma
kidshealth.org/en/kids/asthma.html
Learn more about asthma with this kid-friendly health website.

Respiratory System
kids.britannica.com/kids/article/respiratory-system/353709
Dive deeper into the respiratory system to better understand asthma.

Index